FUNCTIONAL FITNESS ASSESSMENT
FOR
ADULTS OVER 60 YEARS
(A Field Based Assessment)

Second Edition

Wayne H. Osness
Marlene Adrian
Bruce Clark
Werner Hoeger
Diane Raab
Robert Wiswell

Developed by the
Council on Aging and Adult Development
of the
American Association for Active Lifestyles and Fitness

An association of the
American Alliance for Health,
Physical Education, Recreation and Dance

KENDALL/HUNT PUBLISHING COMPANY
4050 Westmark Drive   Dubuque, Iowa 52002

Table of Contents

Preface

The functional fitness assessment of adults over 60 years of age is important to evaluate the ability of the individual to carry on certain daily living activities and even more important as one contemplates a physical training or rehabilitation program intended to help the individual improve their functional capacity over time. The level of fitness not only relates to the ability of the individual to carry on the necessary tasks of daily living but also to maintain the systems of the body that will relate to good health and well being. Clinical assessment has been done for years for the few individuals who have access to medical and allied health facilities that are capable of doing this type of assessment. However, it is also important to provide this functional assessment opportunity for persons over 60 where these facilities are not available.

In 1988, a committee was appointed by the Council of Aging and Adult Development (a structure within the American Association for Active Lifestyles and Fitness) to address the issue of developing a field test that would effectively measure functional fitness in a field setting and without the benefit of highly trained personnel. The American Association for Active Lifestyles and Fitness is an association within the American Alliance for Health, Physical Education, Recreation and Dance. The committee members were Marlene Adrian, PhD., Bruce Clark, PhD., Werner Hoeger, PhD., Wayne Osness, PhD., (Chair), Diane Raab, PhD., and Robert Wiswell, PhD. Ray Ciszek, PhD., was the Alliance Staff Liaison for this committee.

The charge to the committee was to (a) develop an effective field test to determine the functional capacity of older adults, (b) establish age and sex related norms, (c) publish material relative to the test procedures and normative data, (d) establish a training program for professionals in the field using this information, (e) disseminate the test to professionals in the field through various professional channels.

To begin its work the committee reviewed the various assessment procedures in place and the needs for new and better assessment items that were valid and reliable for this population. The committee also identified the target population and the type of tests to be used in the field test situation. The committee then reviewed the locations where such a field test would be conducted and the available personnel at these locations.

Guidelines were then established for the development of a test that would be realistic and still effective in the functional assessment of persons this age. These guidelines were as follows:

1. The test must relate to the full range of age among older people over 60 years. Options may be used for subgroups.

2. The test would not relate to follow-up prescriptions at this point in time.

3. The test would be non diagnostic from a pathological point of view.

4. The test would evaluate the physical function of the older adult.

5. The test would be drug independent.

6. The test will not need physician approval. It will have no more risk than life itself.

7. The test will be prepared for paraprofessional use.

8. The test will require only normally available equipment. No purchased equipment will be necessary.

Because the test was to be a functional fitness test for persons over 60 years of age, it was necessary to establish a working definition of functional fitness. It was decided that functional fitness would be defined as "the physical capacity of the individual to meet ordinary and unexpected demands of daily life safely and effectively." This definition indicated the need for a test that was practical and related closely to activities normally encountered by individuals 60 years of age and above. From the total number of parameters studied in the preliminary testing, a second list of parameters to be included as developed. It included the following: (a) body agility, (b) endurance, (c) flexibility, (d) strength, (e) balance, and (f) coordination.

Test items were then identified having the potential of measuring a given parameter from this list. Each test item was either accepted or rejected due to redundancy or failure to meet the stated guidelines. The previous experience of the committee members as researchers and practitioners in the field was used to prepare this preliminary list of parameters and the selected test items are listed below.

1. Body agility: Agility course

2. Endurance: 880 yard walk, 220 yard walk, 440 yard walk, and 660 yard walk.

3. Flexibility: Sit and reach test, finger touch, and trunk rotation test.

4. Strength: Grip strength, sit/stand test, arm extension with weight, and arm extension at 90° with weight.

5. Balance: One foot stand with eyes open and eyes closed.

6. Coordination: Ruler test and various types of manipulation tests.

The total test structure was then discussed considering the protocols developed, the parameters involved, the items for testing, the scoring procedure, the number of trials to be used, the recording mechanism, and the ability to provide appropriate reliability and validity. The various test items were studied for reliability and validity in the various laboratories of the committee members with validity established by using accepted clinical measures as the standard. At this time body composition was added to the list and both hydrostatic weighting and skin fold formulas used to establish validity.

Validity was established using maximum oxygen intake via treadmill testing for endurance, a variety of clinical flexibility testing procedures for flexibility, clinical isokenetic measurements of a number of muscle groups throughout the body for strength and clinical hand eye coordination measurements for coordination. Quantitative data for reliability can be reviewed within the body of this text. The test-retest method was used to establish reliability values.

The preliminary testing on a larger population provided information on reliability and validity that reduced the number of parameters to the present list. Test protocols were then again revised to the present form. Test items are independent and can be used individually. Only those items should be used that will provide accurate data and will not create unnecessary risk or discomfort for the participant.

The test items included have been tested using a diversified sample of persons over 60 years of age. Items used were found to be reliable and, in some cases, statistically valid for persons of this age.

Population norms have been included in this publication. These norms have been established after several years of testing a large number of persons using the prescribed protocols and testing conditions as outlined in this assessment program. The preliminary testing on the larger population was done to: (1) establish the practicality of the test in a field test situation, (2) provide feedback on the range of discrimination among given age and sex groups, (3) establish preliminary norms, and (4) determine which population this test procedure can most effectively serve.

For development of effective personal assessment procedures for persons over 60 years of age is a continuous process. However, to establish norms that can relate a given individual to standards or to other persons of his or her age and sex requires a collection of a large amount of data using set protocols and conditions for testing. Confusion in the literature often relates to comparing data with similar, but not the same, protocols and varying conditions in testing procedures. The value of the testing program described in this publication is the availability of clear and concise protocols for each of the parameters that can be done in a field test situation, the availability of reliability and validity data that will support the use of these measurement procedures, and a data base that will provide meaningful norms that will provide appropriate feedback to the individuals tested.

1   Introduction

The importance of physical exercise to the older adult has become increasingly apparent during the last decade. Not only does physical exercise improve functional capacity, but evidence is strong that it contributes to an improved health status and a reduction of health related risks. However, the specificity of a given type of exercise and the intensity of that exercise determines the change one can expect to occur in physical function and fitness levels. Change is specific to exercise treatment. This necessitates a careful evaluation of present condition as well as desired outcomes.

Although the opportunity to affect change is great, it is becoming increasingly important to individualize exercise programs and to use the knowledge base available to provide a safe and effective program for the older adult. Therefore, it has become increasingly important that we expand this knowledge base relative to the appropriate amount, duration, and intensity of exercise for a given type of individual, the effects of given types and intensities of activities on a given population, the effect of age and sex, and the consideration of anatomical and physiological limitations of older persons within a given sub group. Although much has been accomplished during the last decade, we still have much to learn to effectively use physical exercise as a means of improving the quality of life for persons over 60 years.

Critical to the expansion of the knowledge base necessary to establish effective exercise programs for the elderly, is the availability of good measuring techniques. First, it is important to effectively assess the condition of a given individual to determine the appropriate exercise prescription that will reduce risk and enhance physiological and psychological change. Secondly, it is important that the measurement techniques are finite enough to quantify change over a period of time to allow for an adjustment in the exercise prescription and thereby enhance the ability of the program to affect long-term change.

Present measurement techniques involve both invasive and non invasive measures, usually performed in a medical setting. These techniques may not be necessary or desirable for the healthy but physically limited individual. Other measurement techniques involve the development of profiles in a clinical setting. These are usual non invasive but involve a considerable amount of equipment and skilled personnel. This type of measurement is often used to assess the effect of a given intervention strategy with relatively small numbers of subjects.

To reach the larger population, it is necessary to have reliable and valid measurement techniques that can be performed by semi-skilled professionals without costly laboratory equipment. Although field-tests are less accurate than clinical or medical measuring techniques, these tests can be used effectively.

Field-tests to assess physical function, or functional fitness among older individuals must be designed for the older population with established reliability and validity for that population. These tests should also relate to the daily function of the individual involved which will ultimately affect the quality of life experienced by that individual. This assessment procedure has been designed to serve the larger population through field based measurement techniques that can be used in a facility where older persons live and can be conducted by personnel not necessarily trained for clinical responsibilities.

2   Rationale for the Test

This assessment program has been designed to use the latest scientific information available as it relates to non invasive assessment of the older adult and the physiological systems that support the physical function of the older adult. It is a functional assessment that can be conducted in a field based setting using large numbers of individuals. Individual results can then be compared to age and sex related norms to assess present condition as well as to assess functional change over time.

When dealing with the older population, one must recognize the increased risk associated with physical activity, particularly during physical assessment when maximal efforts are desired. This test requires a functional maximal performance during which the individual performs to the best of his or her capacity without discomfort or unusual risk. Assessors must recognize that there is a psychological factor related to the intensity of one's performance which will affect and result. However, the individual is expected to perform to the best of his or her ability within the confines of present physical condition. For the older individual, this condition may be affected by several different kinds of anatomical, physiological, or pharmaceutical factors. Although these factors are very important, it is recognized that these same factors would be involved in the development of an exercise prescription designed to enhance physical functionality. The parameters tested and the test items used were selected because each relates to general fitness and the total battery of tests provides a comprehensive evaluation of the individual considering the guidelines previously expressed in this document.

Body composition is measured by ponderal index which involves the relationship between height and weight. The use of anthropometric measurements was discarded because of the need for specific equipment and techniques. In addition, the formulas that use this information to project percent body fat have not been shown effective for older populations. The hydrostatic weighing technique is simply inappropriate for a field-testing situation.

Flexibility is measured by the sit and reach test, which actually measures the flexibility of the lower back and upper leg. The sit and reach test was selected because this test is a reasonable indicator of total body flexibility in the normal older adult. The procedure was

3

developed using a measuring stick to avoid the need for specific equipment that may not be available in a field setting.

Agility and dynamic balance are measured by a new test that involves total body activity. It involves straight ahead movement, change of direction, and changing body position. The test closely relates to the functional movement of the older individual in daily life situations and also provides for a quantitative assessment of this ability. It is the most comprehensive of all test items used in the test battery.

The coordination test also relates to daily function and concentrates on the neuromuscular efficiency of the arms and hands. It is a practical test and one that has good reproducibility as well as finite measurement potential.

Strength was considered an important component of the test battery. The measurement of strength includes an endurance factor using the number of repetitions through a range of motion. The measurement involves the upper body but also has shown good predictability of the total body strength of the older individual. This test was chosen because it was more quantifiable than some of the other field-tests for dynamic strength that are dependent on body weight and moving the body through space.

The endurance test provides a functional assessment of walking ability in older adults. As an assessment of aerobic capacity, validity is moderate but comparable with other walk/run tests based solely on time. The test is highly repeatable after practice in self-pacing. The walk test may be administered in any open, well lighted area with an appropriate surface (even and non slippery).

Each of the test items used is subject to motivation and psychological factors. These factors cannot be totally eliminated in a field-test situation, but care has been taken to provide the test administrator with appropriate directions to standardize the procedure in such a way that the effect of these factors would be minimized.

Prior to the administration of the test, the Exercise/Medical History Form should be used (Section 8) to determine medical and fitness status of the individual. This information can then be used to determine what test protocols are most appropriate for a given individual. Each test parameter is independent, and the clinician can use the information from the form to select the items to be used.

3   Test Items

The test items have complete protocols that must be used for the conduct of the test. Protocols should not be altered in any way so that norms can be used to evaluate the data collected from a given individual and related to a given age and sex cohort group. Each parameter and test item includes the equipment needed, procedure, scoring, trials, and special considerations. The examiner is asked to carefully review the special considerations for the safety of the participant and the validity of the data.

Parameter: Body Composition

Test Item: Ponderal Index

Equipment: Listed under subparameters

Procedure: Body weight and height are determined using procedures detailed in the subparameters below. The measured weight in pounds is placed on the right scale of Figure 3 and measured height is placed on the left scale of Figure 3. A straight line is established using these two points with a straight edge connecting them. The intersection of the center scale provides the reading of Ponderal Index. The higher the Ponderal Index, the greater the degree of leanness.

Scoring: Record Ponderal Index to the nearest .1 of one unit as the score

Trials: Single trial

Subparameter: Body Weight

Test Item: Weight

Equipment: Calibrated scale with increments of 1 lb. or smaller

Procedure: Set the scale on a

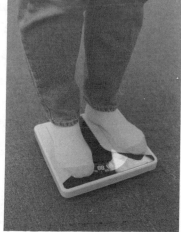

Figure 1.   Weight Measurement

5

firm, flat, horizontal surface. Check that the scale is accurate by using known loads prior to testing. Ask the subject to remove shoes and overgarments, such as coat, jacket, and sweater. Ask the subject to step onto the scale and stand without moving. With subject standing on scale as directed, read the scales to the nearest pound. (Figure 1)

Scoring: Record weight in pounds.

Trials: Single trial

Special Considerations: None

Subparameter: Standing Height Measurement

Test Item: Height

Equipment: Tape measure or other graduated scale of length, masking tape, wall

Procedure: Vertically attach a tape measure to a wall that has no molding strip or other protuberances. Ask the subject to remove shoes, and to turn with back to the wall and place the heels together. Ask the subject to stand erect with head upright and eyes looking straight ahead. With the subject standing as directed, place a flat object, such as a 2" x 4" x 6" wooden block, ruler, or clipboard, horizontally on the top of the crown of the head with one end of the object against the wall. Read the height to the nearest half inch at the intersection of the flat object and the tape measure. If it is difficult to see, ask the subject to stoop slightly and step to one side, but keep the object in place.

(Figure 2)

Scoring: Record height in feet and inches to the nearest half inch.

Trials: One trial

Special Considerations: None

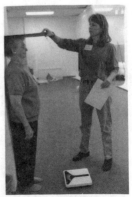

Figure 2. Height Measurement

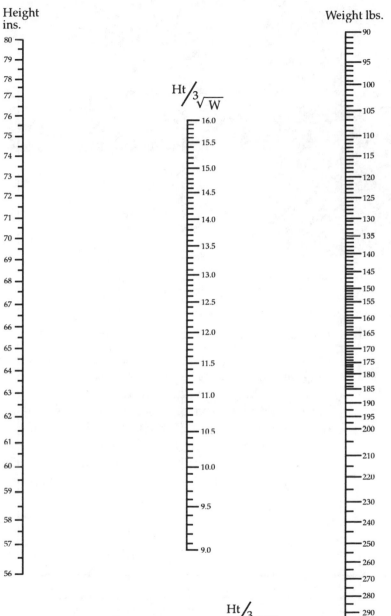

Figure 1. Ponderal Index

$$\text{Ht}\Big/\sqrt[3]{\text{W}}$$

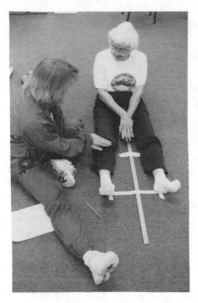

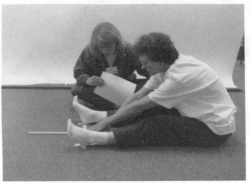

Figure 4. Trunk/Leg Flexibility - Hands should be on top of one another. (Left)

Figure 5. Slide hands forward along the yardstick. (Above)

Parameter: Flexibility

Test Item: Trunk/Leg Flexibility

Equipment: A yardstick, chalk, and masking tape

Set Up: Draw a line or place a piece of masking tape 20" long on the floor. Tape the yardstick to the floor perpendicular to the line with the 25" mark on the yardstick directly over the line. If masking tape is used for the line, the 25" mark should be right at the edge of the tape toward the long end of the yardstick. Next, draw two marks on the line, each 6" away from the center of the yardstick (see Figure 6)

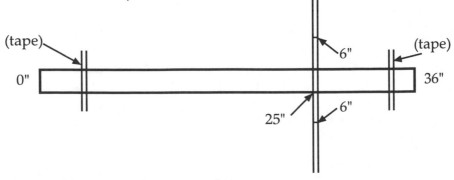

Figure 6. Equipment set-up for the Trunk/Leg Flexibility Test

8

Procedure: The subject should remove shoes for this test, and sit on the floor with legs extended, feet 12" apart, toes pointing straight up, and heels right up against the line (at the 25" mark, and each heel centered at the 6" marks on the line). The yardstick should be between the legs, with the zero point toward the subject. The hands are placed one directly on top of the other. The subject may then slowly reach for ward sliding the hands along the yardstick as far as possible, and must hold the final position for at least 2 seconds. The examiner should place one hand on top of one of the subject's knees to insure that the subject's knees are not raised during the test. (Figures 4 and 5)

Scoring: Record the number of inches reached to the nearest half inch for each trial (.0 or .5). The best trial is recorded as the score.

Trials: Two practice trials followed by two test trials are given. Only the score for the two test trials are recorded.

Approximate Range of Scores: 5" - 30"

Special
Considerations: Be sure that the subjects are properly warmed-up prior to this test. The clinician should use warm-up exercises related to this task. Help all subjects into the sitting position and again when getting up from the floor. The forward reach should be a gradual movement along the top of the yardstick. The tip of the middle fingers must remain even during the entire reaching action, and the final position must be held for at least 2 seconds. Be sure that the toes are straight up and that the legs are kept as straight as possible. If feet start turning outward or the knees start to come up during the reaching action, ask the subject to maintain the correct position.

9

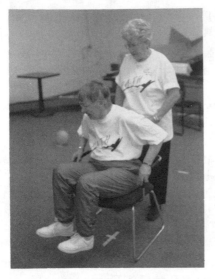
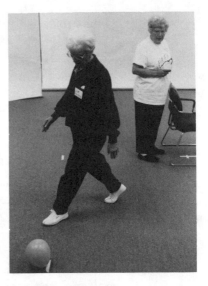

Figure 7. Agility/Dynamic Balance –
Use your hands to get up from the chair.

Figure 8. Walk as fast as is comfortable.

Parameter: Agility/Dynamic Balance

Test Item: Agility/Dynamic Balance

Equipment: Chair with arms (average seat height: 16"), mask
ing or duct tape, measuring tape, two cones, stop
watch

Set Up: The initial placement of the chair should be marked
with the legs taped to the floor, or held to avoid moving during the test. Measuring from the spot on the
floor (X) in front of the chair where the feet will be
placed, the cones are set up with their farthest edge
located 6' to the side and 5' behind the initial mea-

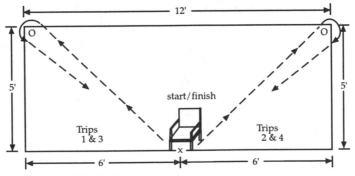

Figure 9. Diagram of Agility Course

suring spot (X). One cone is set up at either side behind the chair (see Figure 9). The area should be well lit, the floor even and nonslippery. Arrows should be placed on the floor in appropriate locations to remind the subjects of the proper pathway.

Procedure: The subject begins fully seated in the chair with heels on the ground. On the signal "Ready, go," the subject stands up from the chair, moves to the right, going to the inside and around the back of the cone (counterclockwise), (Figure 8), returns directly to the chair, sits down, and raises the feet 1/2" from the floor, (Figure 7). With out hesitating, the subject gets up immediately, moves to the left, again going to the inside and around the back of the cone (clock wise), returns di rectly to the chair, sits down com pleting one circuit. The subject stands up immedi ately and repeats a second circuit exactly as the first. One trial consists of two complete circuits (going around the cones four times [right, left, right, left]).

During the test, after circling the cones, the subject must sit down fully in the chair. This means the subject must lift the feet 1/2" from the floor before standing up. The subject must use his or her hands to get in and out of the chair. Subjects should go as fast as they feel comfortable without losing their balance or falling.

Explain the test procedure, then walk the subject through the course to make sure he or she circles the cones correctly and that subjects lift their feet each time they sit down. Give the following instructions to the subject: "Walk (do not run) as fast as comfortable without feeling you will lose your balance or fall. One trial consists of circling each cone two times. The first time, go to your right, then to your left, right, and left. Go around the cone from the inside to the outside. Come back and sit down after circling each cone. Sit down fully and lift your feet off the floor each time. Use your hands to help you get in and out of the chair without falling. If you feel dizzy, light headed, or you notice any pain, stop immediately and tell me."

During the test give verbal directions (e.g. right, left, around, sit down, etc.) so the subject does not have to stop or hesitate because he or she is confused. Make sure the subjects lift their feet each time they sit down. If the subject moves the chair, the technician should readjust it to the original position during the trial.

Trials: A practice "walk through" should be administered until the subject demonstrates that he or she understands the test. Two trials are administered with 30 seconds rest provided after each trial.

Score: Record the time for each trial to the nearest 0.1 seconds. The best trial is recorded as the score.

Approximate Range of Scores: Most people will score between 15 - 35 seconds.

Parameter: Coordination

Test Item: "Soda Pop" Coordination Test.

Equipment: Three unopened (12 oz.) cans of soda pop, a stop watch, 3/4" masking tape, a table, and a chair.

Set Up: Using the 3/4" masking tape, place a 30" strip of tape on the table, about 5" from the edge of the table. Draw six marks exactly 5" away from each other along the line of tape, starting at 2 1/2" away from either edge of the tape. Now place six strips of tape, each 3" long, centered exactly on top of each of the six marks previously drawn. For the purpose of this test, each little "square" formed by the crossing of the long strip of tape and the 3" strip of tape is assigned a number starting with 1 for the first square on the right to 6 for the last square on the left. (Figure 10)

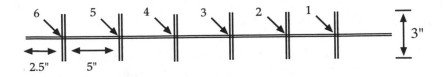

Figure 10. Masking Tape Placement for the "Soda Pop" Coordination Test

Procedure: To administer the test, have the subject sit comfort ably in front of the table, the body centered with the diagram on the table. The preferred hand is used for this test. If the right hand is used, place three cans of soda pop on the table in the following manner: Can #1 is centered on square 1 (farthest to the right), can #2 on square 3, and can #3 on square 5. To start the test, the right hand, with the thumb up, is placed on can #1 and the elbow joint should be at about 100-120°. When the examiner gives the signal, the stopwatch is started and the subject pro ceeds to turn the cans of pop upside down, placing can #1 over square 2, (Figure 11), followed by can #2 over square 4, and then can #3 over square 6. (Figure 12)

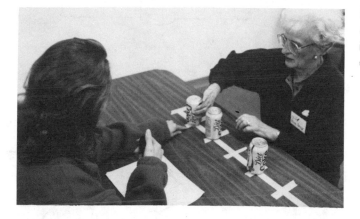

Figure 11. Coor-dination - Can #1 is turned upside down.

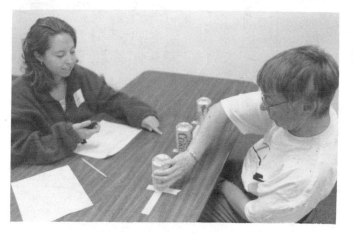

Figure 12. On "return trip" cans are grasped with the thumb down.

Immediately, the subject returns all three cans starting with can #1, then can #2, and can #3, returning them to their original placement. On this "return trip," the cans are grasped with the hand in a thumb down position. This entire procedure is done twice, without stopping, and counted as one trial. In other words, two "trips" down and up are required to complete one trial. The watch is stopped when the last can is returned to its original position, following the second trip back. The preferred hand (in this case, the right hand) is used throughout the entire task (a graphic illustration of this test is provided in Figure 13). The object of the test is to

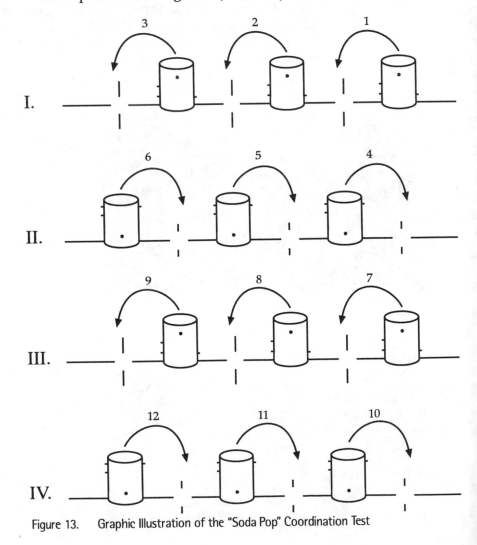

Figure 13. Graphic Illustration of the "Soda Pop" Coordination Test

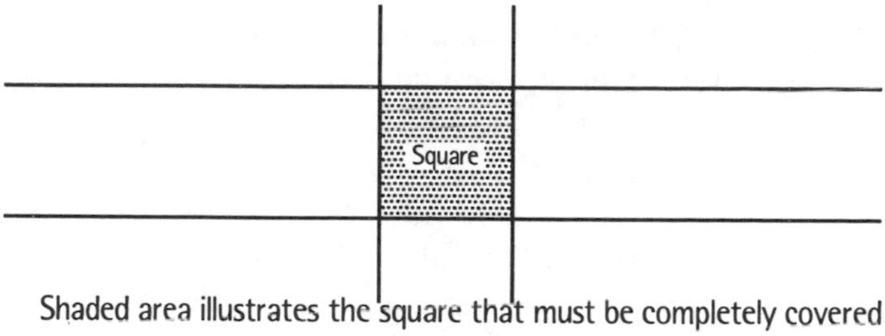

Figure 14.   Shaded area illustrates the square that must be completely covered when turning the cans during the "Soda Pop" Coordination Test

perform the task as fast as possible, making sure that the cans are always placed over the squares. If a can misses a square at any time during the test, the trial must be repeated from the start. A miss indicates that a can did not completely cover the entire square formed by the crossing of the two strips of tape (see Figure 14).

If a participant chooses to use the left hand, the same procedures are used, except that the cans are placed starting from the left, with can #1 over square 6, can #2 over square 4, and can #3 over square 2. The procedure is initiated by turning can #1 upside down over square 5, can #2 onto square 3, etc.

Scoring: Record the time of each test trial to the nearest 0.1 of a second.

Trials: Two practice trials followed by two test trials are given. Only the scores for the two test trials are recorded. The best trial is recorded as the score.

Approximate Range of Scores: 8 - 25 seconds

Special Considerations: During the entire procedure, the cans must completely cover the squares formed by the crossing of the two tapes. If the subject has a mistrial (misses a square), repeat the test until two successful trials are accomplished.

Parameter: Strength/Endurance

Test Item: Strength/Endurance Test

Equipment: Four and eight lb. weights, or a 1/2 gal. plastic milk bottle with handle and a one gallon plastic

15

milk bottle with handle, sand, water, or other similar material, stopwatch, normal chair without arms, (4 and 8 lb. weights are optional).

Set Up: As an alternative to weights, a 1/2 gal. empty milk bottle should be filled with sand, water, or other material to 4 lbs. of total weight and the cover tightened. A 1 gal. empty milk bottle can then be filled in the same way to 8 lbs. and the cover tightened. Four and eight pound hand weights are to be used if available and weighed for accuracy. A straight backed chair with no arms is placed in an area with no obstructions.

Procedures: The subject is asked to sit in a chair with the back straight and against the back of the chair as much as possible. The subject's eyes should be looking straight ahead and the feet should be flat on the floor in a comfortable position. The nondominant hand should be resting in the lap with the dominant arm hanging to the side. The subject's arm should be straight and relaxed.

The weight or weighted milk bottle is placed thumbs up, in the dominant hand that is extended toward the floor. The subject is asked to grasp the handle and hold it in the extended position. The 4 lb. weight (1/2 gal. container) should be used for women and the 8 lb. weight (one gallon container) should be used for men. The running stopwatch should be placed in the nondominant hand resting in the lap and facing the dominant side of the body. The examiner should stand on the side of the subject's dominant arm and place one hand on the dominant biceps, helping to support the weight with the other hand. The hand helping to support the milk bottle is then removed and the subject is asked to contract the biceps through the full range of motion until the lower arm touches the hand of the examiner on the biceps, (Figure 15). This represents one total repetition. If the subject cannot bring the weight through the full range of motion, the test is terminated with a score of zero.

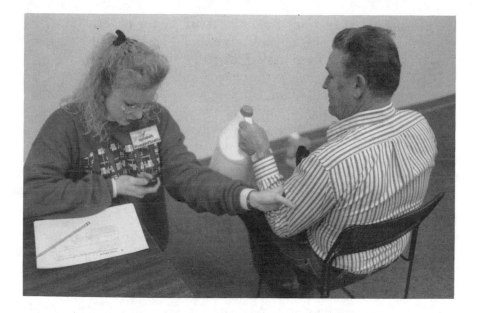

Figure 15. Strength/Endurance – Contract the biceps through the full range of motion until the lower arm touches the hand of the examiner.

When the practice repetition is complete, the weight is placed on the floor for approximately 1 minute and again placed in the hand supported by the examiner. The examiner then instructs the subject to make as many repetitions as possible in 30 seconds. The lower arm must touch the examiner's hand (on the biceps) and be completely extended for a complete repetition. While watching the stopwatch, the examiner instructs the subject to begin (unassisted) and counts the num ber of repetitions the subject can do in the 30-second period. The examiner starts and stops the time interval at a convenient time on the stopwatch.

Trials: One 30-second trial.

Scoring: Record the maximal number of complete repetitions in the 30-second interval.

Range of Scores: 0 - 40 repetitions

Special
Considerations: If the subject cannot grasp the handle of the weight to hold it in place, this test should not be used.Subjects should be instructed to breathe normally during the test. The weight

should not be bounced off the floor. If this is the case, elevate the chair. Subjects should be instructed to stop the test if the subject experiences pain in the tested arm. The examiner must determine if the pain is due to a structural condition or lack of strength. If the former, the test will be invalid and no score recorded.

Parameter: Endurance

Test Item: 880 Yard Walk

Equipment: Stopwatch, measuring tape, cones

Set-Up: The test involves a continuous walk of 880 yards. The subject will walk around a measured lap until he or she has walked a total of 880 yards. Using a measuring tape or similar device, measure an oval lap as large as possible, and compute the number of laps required to complete 880 yards. Mark the inside edges of the lap (oval or rectangle) with the cones. The lap should be designed with sufficient space to make a turn, reducing the effects of a quick change in direction. The area will be well lit, the surface nonslippery and level. All obstacles should be removed from the path. People not taking the test should not be allowed to walk onto the course during the test.

Procedure: Instruct the subject to walk the course (x number of laps) as fast as he or she feels comfortable. Subjects may not run. They should walk at their own pace independent of the other participants. Do not allow people to walk in pairs or groups. It is important they pace themselves so they are able to finish the distance and do not experience discomfort. If a person is dizzy, lightheaded, nauseous, or experiences any pain, he or she should stop the test immediately and inform the examiner. On the signal, "Ready, go," the subject begins at a designated spot and walks the necessary laps until he or she reaches 880 yards. (Figures 16 and 17)

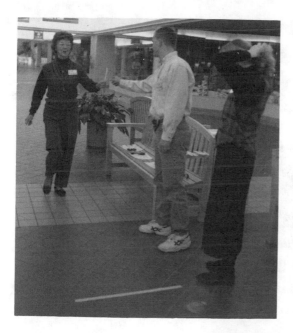

Figure 16. Endurance - Walk a measured course of 880 yards.

Figure 17. Endurance - A "popsicle stick" is given as each lap is completed to keep track of total number of laps.

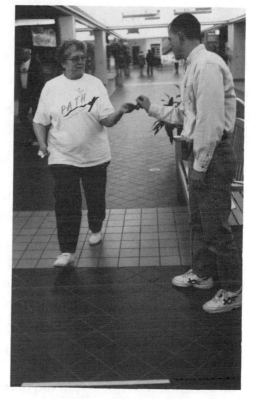

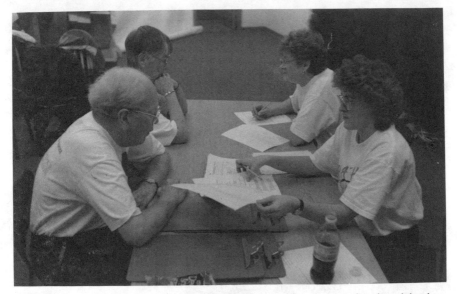

Figure 18.   Consent and Medical History Forms should be completed and explained to participants.

Trials: A single trial is used.

Score: Record the time in minutes and seconds to the nearest second as the score.

Approximate Range of Scores: 5 minutes to 14 minutes 30 seconds

Special   Screen individuals for cardiovascular or orthopedic contraindications, (Figure 18). Under the following circumstances the examiner should either discourage or not allow the participants to perform the test without first consulting their physician:

a.   Significant orthopedic problems that may be aggravated by prolonged continuous walking (8-10 minutes).

b.   History of cardiac problems (i.e., recent heart attack, fre quent arrhythmia, valvular defects) that can be negatively influenced by exertion.

c.   Lightheadedness upon activity or history of uncontrolled hypertension (high blood pres sure).

The walk test should be administered last in the battery of tests. The warm-up session is left to the discretion of the examiner. Individuals should practice walking several days prior to the test to determine an appropriate walking pace.

4. Reliability and Validity of the Test Items

During the development of the battery of test, and particularly during the selection of test items, it was necessary to establish reliability and validity values for the test items and protocols proposed. Several trail protocols were developed for each of the parameters selected. Each trail protocol was tested to establish levels of reliability and validity. Those protocols that had the best reliability and validity values were then selected to be used in the test battery for that parameter.

Table I shows the results of the reliability studies completed for each of the parameters used in the field test. In most cases, reliability studies were done in multiple laboratories directed by members of the committee. The test pre-test method was used for reliability and each of the final test items were found to have acceptable reliability. Care was taken to ensure the fact that all data was collected using controlled conditions and exactly the same testing procedure. This data indicates that the day to day variation is very small for these test items and that a given subject will provide very similar data from one test session to another. This was important to the committee because of the concern that a functional test is not necessarily a maximal test. Often a maximal test will provide greater reliability than a functional test.

Table II provides similar data for the establishment of validity. Ponderal index, the sit and reach test and the agility course test items do not have a clinical equivalent and therefore a standard that is accepted by the profession. As a result, it was necessary for the committee to use its best judgment concerning the validity of these particular items to provide quality data for the given parameter. The "soda pop" test for hand eye coordination was validated using typical laboratory procedures for reaction time, hand steadiness, hand eye coordination, and hand eye coordination. Theses coefficients were relatively low. However, this test item gave the best values of any that were tried for this parameter. One will also note that the number of subjects used was 90. The arm curl was validated using a cybex protocol elbow curl and the correlation was considerably higher. However, it must be noted that the number of subjects was

TABLE I
AAHPERD Field Test Battery
"Functional Fitness Assessment
For Adults Over 60 Years"

PARAMETER	TEST ITEM	RELIABILITY STUDY	GENDER (n)	r
Body Composition	Ponderal Index	Osness (1990)	Men and Women (84)	0.994
Flexibility	Sit and Reach	Wiswell(1990)	Men (75)	0.988-0.991
			Women (75)	0.978-0.99
Agility/Dynamic	Agility Course	Hoeger (1990)	Men and Women (14)	0.99
Balance		Osness (1990)	Men and Women (14)	0.995
		Wiswell (1990)	Men (72)	0.963-0.986
			Women (260)	0.947-0.978
Coordination	Soda Pop	Hoeger (1990)	Men (15)	0.911
		Raab (1990)	Women (30)	0.853 -0.911
		Wiswell (1990)	Men (75)	0.958-0.993
			Women (285)	0.929-0.955
		Hoeger (1990)	Men and Women Rt. (14)	0.93
				0.86
			Men and Women Lt. (14)	
Strength/	Arm Curl	Burdsall (1991)	Men and Women (13)	0.833
Endurance		Osness (1991)	Men and Women (28)	0.927
		Wiswell (1990)	Men (42)	0.884-0.947
			Women (105)	0.807-0.931
		Osness (1990)	Men (36)	0.921
			Women (64)	0.894
Endurance	800 yd Walk	Raab (1990)	Men (15)	0.82

also much lower. The endurance test using the 800 yard walk was done by using measurement of maximal oxygen intake per minute. This was done on the treadmill and using laboratory controlled conditions. The end point of the test was determined using ACSM guidelines. Shorter endurance walks were studied but did not provide validity values that were acceptable. It was decided that it would be better not to use a given test item than to accept validity values that were lower than the 0.615. This level could only be achieved using the 880 yard walk.

Several other studies have been published relating to the reliability and/or validity of the test items used. These studies support the relative levels of reliability and validity found in the initial study of the test items. (See the list of suggested resources/ references).

TABLE II
AAPHERD Field Test Battery
"Functional Fitness Assessment
For Adults Over 60 Years"

AAHPERD TEST ITEM	LABORATORY STANDARD	CORRELATION COEFFICIENT	SUBJECTS n
Ponderal Index	None	Assumed	-
Sit and Reach	None	Assumed	-
Agility Course	None	Assumed	-
Soda Pop	Reaction Time	0.59	90
	Hand Steadiness	0.399	90
	Eye-Hand Coord.	0.349	90
Arm Curl	Cybex Elbow Curl	0.82	7
800yd Walk	VO2 max	0.615	15

5   Age And Gender Related Norms and Performance Levels

Since, 1990, data has been collected using these test items and protocols to evaluate the functional fitness of individuals over 60 years of age. Data from over 2,000 individuals has been collected to be used to establish norms for age and sex related cohort groups. The data collected is a random sample and good cross section of individuals of this age that are ambulatory and are able to complete the test protocols. The age groups were divided into five year intervals and evaluated for both males and females. The number of individuals in each of these subgroups (count) varies because of the larger number of individuals in the lower age groups and the larger number of females that have been tested. It is also important to note that not all of the test items were used for each person tested. The test items and protocols have been developed to be independent, test items have been treated separately and the performance on one test is not affected by the others. All of those tested did not complete the total test battery.

It should be noted that the performance levels of age and gender subgroups do not necessarily decline with age in all of the test items used to establish performance norms. It is also important to note that the variance in a given test item and at a given age or gender subgroup varies as well.

The norms were established by calculating the mean and standard deviation for the data collected in each of the age and sex subgroups. The performance levels were determined by using the standard deviations and considering the performance of individuals above one standard deviation from the mean to be above average, those below one standard deviation from the mean to be below average and those individuals within one standard deviation of the mean to be average. This is an arbitrary performance evaluation and can be adjusted to the needs of the person using the test results. However, it does give an indication of how an individual relates to his or her age and sex cohorts. It is important to note that the numbers used are actual data and therefore do not represent a linear regression of performance by the range of age groups. It should also be noted that the variance, as determined by the standard deviation, could indicate that there is no significant performance differences from one age group to the next. Again, the user can apply this data to the individual as he or she feels it would best describe the performance level in an applied situation.

Ponderal Index is an established relationship between height and weight. The test protocol indicates the procedures used to establish Ponderal Index (P.I.). This is a general indication of body composition. The greater the P.I., the greater the leanness of the individual as compared to his or her height. One can quickly observe that there is only modest variation among the age and gender subgroups.

Flexibility was measured in inches and tenths of inches with the greater number of inches the higher functional level. It can be noted that there is a decline in mean values with age and the female mean values were higher than the male mean values.

The agility/balance was measured in seconds and tenths of seconds. The lower the number of seconds, the greater the performance level. The norms indicate a decline in performance with age with a similar trend for males and females.

Coordination was measured by a timed performance in seconds and tenths of seconds. Performance levels were greater as the number of seconds declined. There is a modest decline in performance level with age and very little difference between males and females.

Strength/endurance was measured by the number of repetitions within a thirty second interval. The greater number of repetitions represented the higher performance level. A considerable decline in performance occurred with age in this test item.. However, only a slight difference was noted between males and females.

Endurance was measured in minutes and hundredths of minutes of the timed endurance walk. As the number of minutes declined, the performance level improved. A considerable decline in performance occurred with advanced age and the mean values for men were consistently lower than the mean values for women. It must be noted that the data collected during the test procedure was in minutes and seconds. It was necessary to convert the minutes and seconds to minutes and hundredths of minutes for effective statistical evaluation. In an applied setting it would be appropriate to simply estimate the decimal equivalent of the minute as related to the number of seconds in the actual score. For example, thirty seconds would be equivalent to .50 hundredths of a minute. The reason for this conversion is that normal stop watches measure in minutes and seconds and typical statistical analysis must be done in decimal equivalents.

Table III through Table XX provide age and gender related norms as well as performance levels for each of the six parameters. The age and gender related performance levels are not intended to closely discriminate among individuals but simply to relate those performances that are average, above average, or below average. Most individuals will fall into the average group. The clinician can adjust these values in any way that he or she feels most appropriate. The count for each of the age and sex groups provides the user with an opportunity to appropriately evaluate the application of these numbers to the applied situation.

TABLE III
Age and Gender Related Norms
Ponderal Index
(Measured in P. I. Units)

Age Range	Men			Women		
	Mean	Standard Deviation	Count	Mean	Standard Deviation	Count
60-64	11.92	0.44	96	11.69	0.80	225
65-69	11.89	0.48	120	11.82	0.81	285
70-74	12.03	0.64	84	11.83	0.77	315
75-79	11.93	0.64	102	11.92	0.69	330
80-84	11.61	0.55	51	11.64	0.95	201
85-90	11.88	0.68	30	12.01	0.80	61

TABLE IV
Age Related Performance Levels for
Ponderal Index for Men
(Measured in P. I. Units)

Age Range	Above Average	Average	Below Average
60-64	Above 12.36	12.36-11.48	Below 11.48
65-69	Above 12.37	12.37-11.41	Below 11.41
70-74	Above 12.67	12.67-11.39	Below 11.39
75-79	Above 12.57	12.57-11.29	Below 11.29
80-84	Above 12.16	12.16-11.06	Below 11.06
85-90	Above 12.56	12.56-11.20	Below 11.20

TABLE V
Age Related Performance Levels for
Ponderal Index for Women
(Measured in P. I. Units)

Age Range	Above Average	Average	Below Average
60-64	Above 12.49	12.49-10.89	Below 10.89
65-69	Above 12.63	12.63-11.01	Below 11.01
70-74	Above 12.60	12.60-11.06	Below 11.06
75-79	Above 12.61	12.61-11.23	Below 11.23
80-84	Above 12.89	12.89-10.99	Below 10.99
85-90	Above 12.81	12.81-12.01	Below 12.01

TABLE VI
Age and Gender Related Norms
Flexibility
(Measured in inches and tenths of inches)

Age Range	Men			Women		
	Mean	Standard Deviation	Count	Mean	Standard Deviation	Count
60-64	19.90	5.00	40	23.23	5.02	113
65-69	19.84	5.04	69	23.60	6.17	152
70-74	17.86	6.11	60	22.60	5.75	139
75-79	18.53	5.59	48	22.91	6.32	135
80-84	18.37	3.95	20	20.88	5.89	77
85-90	16.20	2.82	15	19.53	6.21	38

TABLE VII
Age Related Performance Levels for
Flexibility for Men
(Measured in inches and tenths of inches)

Age Range	Above Average	Average	Below Average
60-64	Above 24.90	24.90-14.90	Below 14.90
65-69	Above 24.88	24.88-14.80	Below 14.80
70-74	Above 23.97	23.97-11.75	Below 11.75
75-79	Above 24.12	24.12-12.94	Below 12.94
80-84	Above 22.32	22.32-14.42	Below 14.42
85-90	Above 19.02	19.02-13.38	Below 13.38

TABLE VIII
Age Related Performance Levels for
Flexibility for Women
(Measured in inches and tenths of inches)

Age Range	Above Average	Average	Below Average
60-64	Above 28.25	28.25-18.21	Below 18.21
65-69	Above 29.72	29.72-17.43	Below 17.43
70-74	Above 28.35	28.35-16.85	Below 16.85
75-79	Above 29.23	29.23-16.59	Below 16.59
80-84	Above 26.77	26.77-14.99	Below 14.99
85-90	Above 25.74	25.74-13.32	Below 13.32

TABLE IX
Age and Gender Related Norms
Agility/Balance
(Measured in seconds and tenths of seconds)

Age Range	Men			Women		
	Mean	Standard Deviation	Count	Mean	Standard Deviation	Count
60-64	25.36	6.14	55	24.97	5.43	207
65-69	26.49	8.03	98	27.37	6.24	336
70-74	28.21	13.10	80	29.04	7.05	289
75-79	31.75	8.33	57	34.02	10.62	235
80-84	32.60	9.25	23	37.09	15.10	96
85-90	33.56	16.49	13	42.25	15.66	32

TABLE X
Age Related Performance Levels for
Agility/Balance for Men
(Measured in seconds and tenths of seconds)

Age Range	Above Average	Average	Below Average
60-64	Below 19.22	19.22-31.50	Above 31.50
65-69	Below 18.46	18.46-34.52	Above 34.52
70-74	Below 15.11	15.11-41.31	Above 41.31
75-79	Below 23.42	23.42-40.08	Above 40.08
80-84	Below 23.35	23.35-41.85	Above 41.85
85-90	Below 17.07	17.07-50.05	Above 50.05

TABLE XI
Age Related Performance Levels for
Agility/Balance for Women
(Measured in seconds and tenths of seconds)

Age Range	Above Average	Average	Below Average
60-64	Below 19.54	19.54-30.40	Above 30.40
65-69	Below 21.13	21.13-33.61	Above 33.61
70-74	Below 21.99	21.99-36.09	Above 36.09
75-79	Below 23.40	23.40-44.64	Above 44.64
80-84	Below 21.99	21.99-52.19	Above 52.19
85-90	Below 26.59	26.59-57.91	Above 57.91

TABLE XII
Age and Gender Related Norms
Coordination
(Measured in seconds and tenths of seconds)

Age Range	Men			Women		
	Mean	Standard Deviation	Count	Mean	Standard Deviation	Count
60-64	11.66	2.68	58	12.12	3.20	155
65-69	12.48	2.35	87	12.61	3.43	182
70-74	13.04	3.53	70	12.93	3.73	191
75-79	13.45	2.37	59	13.56	4.57	194
80-84	14.22	3.13	26	14.54	3.80	92
85-90	13.57	3.40	16	15.68	3.27	35

TABLE XIII
Age Related Performance Levels for
Coordination for Men
(Measured in seconds and tenths of seconds)

Age Range	Above Average	Average	Below Average
60-64	Below 8.98	8.98-14.34	Above 14.34
65-69	Below 10.13	10.13-14.83	Above 14.83
70-74	Below 9.51	9.51-16.57	Above 16.57
75-79	Below 11.08	11.08-15.82	Above 15.82
80-84	Below 11.09	11.09-17.35	Above 17.35
85-90	Below 10.17	10.17-16.97	Above 16.97

TABLE XIV
Age Related Performance Levels for
Coordination for Women
(Measured in seconds and tenths of seconds)

Age Range	Above Average	Average	Below Average
60-64	Below 8.92	8.92-15.31	Above 15.31
65-69	Below 9.18	9.18-16.04	Above 16.04
70-74	Below 9.20	9.20-16.66	Above 16.66
75-79	Below 8.99	8.99-18.13	Above 18.13
80-84	Below 10.74	10.74-18.34	Above 18.34
85-90	Below 12.41	12.41-18.95	Above 18.95

TABLE XV
Age and Gender Related Norms
Strength/Endurance
(Measured in repetitions)

Age Range	Men			Women		
	Mean	Standard Deviation	Count	Mean	Standard Deviation	Count
60-64	23.69	5.46	58	21.78	6.20	126
65-69	21.47	6.91	92	21.21	6.73	146
70-74	21.14	5.76	74	20.79	6.06	147
75-79	20.15	4.09	65	17.70	5.17	149
80-84	20.53	2.61	30	17.59	4.89	95
85-90	17.82	5.10	22	16.20	4.77	41

TABLE XVI
Age Related Performance Levels for
Strength/Endurance for Men
(Measured in repetitions)

Age Range	Above Average	Average	Below Average
60-64	Above 29.15	29.15-18.23	Below 18.23
65-69	Above 28.38	28.38-14.56	Below 14.56
70-74	Above 26.90	26.90-15.38	Below 15.38
75-79	Above 24.24	24.24-16.06	Below 16.06
80-84	Above 23.14	23.14-17.92	Below 17.92
85-90	Above 22.92	22.92-12.72	Below 12.72

TABLE XVII
Age Related Performance Levels for
Strength/Endurance for Women
(Measured in repetitions)

Age Range	Above Average	Average	Below Average
60-64	Above 27.98	27.98-15.58	Below 15.58
65-69	Above 27.94	27.94-14.48	Below 14.48
70-74	Above 26.85	26.85-14.73	Below 14.73
75-79	Above 22.87	22.87-12.53	Below 12.53
80-84	Above 22.48	22.48-12.70	Below 12.70
85-90	Above 20.97	20.97-11.43	Below 11.43

TABLE XVIII
Age and Gender Related Norms
Endurance
(Measured in minutes and hundredths of minutes)

Age Range	Men Mean	Men Standard Deviation	Men Count	Women Mean	Women Standard Deviation	Women Count
60-64	7.12	1.28	33	8.44	1.56	148
65-69	7.82	1.52	80	8.96	2.07	220
70-74	8.34	1.27	67	9.09	2.37	168
75-79	9.73	3.74	44	9.97	1.87	145
80-84	8.09	1.40	14	10.71	2.35	53
85-90	9.52	1.37	11	10.38	2.10	22

TABLE IXX
Age Related Performance Levels for
Endurance for Men
(Measured in minutes and hundredths of minutes)

Age Range	Above Average	Average	Below Average
60-64	Below 5.84	5.84-8.40	Above 8.40
65-69	Below 6.30	6.30-9.34	Above 9.34
70-74	Below 7.07	7.07-9.61	Above 9.61
75-79	Below 5.99	5.99-13.47	Above 13.47
80-84	Below 6.69	6.69-9.49	Above 9.49
85-90	Below 8.15	8.15-10.89	Above 10.89

TABLE XX
Age Related Performance Levels for
Endurance for Women
(Measured in minutes and hundredths of minutes)

Age Range	Above Average	Average	Below Average
60-64	Below 6.88	6.88-10.00	Above 10.00
65-69	Below 6.69	6.69-10.83	Above 10.83
70-74	Below 6.72	6.72-11.46	Above 11.46
75-79	Below 8.10	8.10-11.84	Above 11.84
80-84	Below 8.36	8.36-13.06	Above 13.06
85-90	Below 8.28	8.28-12.48	Above 12.48

6   Test Results Application

The use of the functional fitness test and norms can vary as determined by the user. However, the test was designed to assist the user to (1) evaluate change with intervention strategies, (2) establish the condition of the individual prior to preparing an exercise prescription, and (3) provide feedback to the individual about his or her functional capacity. This information can also be used to establish the ability of a given individual to effectively and safely complete necessary self care responsibilities and living arrangements. In this case, it would probably be one of several measures that will contribute to the decision making process.

Motivation is one of the major problems as we address the importance of regular exercise to the health and well being of the person over 60 years of age. Hopefully, feedback of this nature will help to provide motivation to continue the exercise program and demonstrate that the appropriate type of exercise program will provide predictable outcomes. Motivation may also be enhanced through various kinds of award systems that will recognize achievement and a sense of pride in one's accomplishments.

The development of intervention strategies to improve the physical function of the adult over 60 years must be done using as much data as possible to maximize the effect of that intervention strategy and establish a reasonable level of safety. Performance test data will provide an indication of the functional capacity of the individual and the level of intensity that will best reflect the needs of that individual. The national norms provided in this publication can be used for this assessment. However, it may be that the user would like to establish local norms that relate to a specific population. In either case, the information can effectively be used to develop intervention strategies that are both safe and effective.

Computer software is also available that will provide immediate feedback on the performance levels of individuals as compared to national norms. However, this too can be done at the local level as well. This software can graphically provide information to individuals that relates to strengths and weaknesses in functional performance as compared to others of the same age and sex. The profile is a more accurate comparison of the individual to others of the same age and sex that have been tested. The profile will also assist the clinician in the evaluation of the results of this assessment and the development of individualized intervention strategies. The reader can contact the University of Kansas Fitness Clinic, Department of Health, Physical Education and Recreation, University of Kansas, Lawrence, KS 66045 for more information concerning the profile software and the availability of profiles from a given data set.

7

Data Sheet

FUNCTIONAL FITNESS ASSESSMENT FOR ADULTS OVER 60 YEARS
INDIVIDUAL DATA COLLECTION FORM

Name _____ Testing Date _____   D/M/Y _____

Sex: F M   Age: ____ yrs.   Location: _____

Test Administrator: _____

Administer the 5 item test battery in the suggested sequence. (Endurance Walk and Agility/Dynamic Balance tests should not be given consecutively.)

Test Item		Test Trials/Score		
		Trial 1	Trial 2	Final Recorded Score
1. Ponderal Index (to nearest .1 of Unit)				
	Weight [ ][ ] [ ].[ ] lb.			
	Height [ ] [ ].[ ] in.			
	Ponderal Index [ ] [ ].[ ] Units			
2. Flexibility (score to .5 inch) Practice given, not recorded.		[ ][ ].[ ]	[ ][ ].[ ]	[ ][ ].[ ]
3. Agility/Dynamic Balance - Score seconds & tenths of seconds.		[ ][ ].[ ]	[ ][ ].[ ]	[ ][ ].[ ]
4. Coordination - Score seconds & tenths of seconds. Practice given, not recorded.		[ ][ ].[ ]	[ ][ ].[ ] [ ][ ].[ ]	[ ][ ].[ ]
5. Strength - Score # of repetitions in 30 sec. 4# Women. 8# Men (single lift practice)				[ ][ ]
6. Endurance Walk - Time in minutes and seconds			[ ][ ].[ ][ ]	[ ][ ].[ ]

Note: Convert to seconds and tenths of seconds to use profile and norms.

8 Exercise/Medical History Form

MEDICAL/EXERCISE ASSESSMENT FOR OLDER ADULTS

Name _____ Phone _____ Date _____
Street _____ City _____ State ___ Zip _____

PART I - TO BE FILLED OUT BY PARTICIPANT

A. ACTIVITY HISTORY

1. How would you rate your physical activity level during the last year?

___ LITTLE - Sitting, typing, driving, talking - NO planned exercise

___ MILD - Standing, walking, bending, reaching

___ MODERATE - Standing, walking bending, reaching, exercise 1 day a week

___ ACTIVE - Light physical work, climbing stairs, exercise 2-3 days a week

___ VERY ACTIVE - Moderate physical work, regular exercise 4 or more days a week

2. What exercise and recreational activities are you presently involved in and how often? _____

B. HEALTH HISTORY

Weight _____ Height _____ Recent weight loss/gain _____
Please list any recent illnesses: _____

Please list hospitalizations and reasons during last 5 years: _____

PLEASE CHECK THE BOX IN FRONT OF THOSE QUESTIONS TO WHICH YOUR ANSWER IS YES:

_Anemia

_Arthritis/Bursitis

_Asthma

_Blood pressure _____

_Bowel/Bladder problems

_Chest pains

_Chest discomfort while exercising

_Diabetes

_Difficulty with hearing _____

_Difficulty with vision _____

_Dizziness or balance problems

_Heart conditions _____

_Hernia

_Indigestion

_Joint pain in _____

_Leg pain on walking

_Lung disease

_Shortness of breath

_Passing out spells

_Osteoporosis _____

_Low back condition

_Other orthopedic conditions (list)

SMOKING: Never smoked   Smoke now (how much?___)   Smoked in past

ALCOHOL CONSUMPTION: None   Occasional   Often (how much?_____)

List any existing health concerns: _____

Please list medications and/or dietary supplements you regularly take: _____

PART II — TO BE FILLED OUT BY PHYSICIAN-DATE OF LAST EXAM _____
A. PHYSICAL EXAMINATION — Please check if it applies to the patient.

_Resting heart rate _____   _Resting blood pressure _____
_Chest auscultation abnormal   _Thyroid abnormal
_Heart size abnormal   _Any joints abnormal
_Peripheral pulses normal   _Abnormal masses
_Abnormal heart sounds, gallops   _Other _____

PRESENT PRESCRIBED MEDICATION(S)_____

B. CARDIOVASCULAR LABORATORY EXAMINATION (Within one year of the present date if recommended by physician)
DATE: _____

Resting ECG: Rate _____ Rhythm _____

Axis _____ Interpretation _____

Stress Test: Max H.R. _____ Max B.P. _____ Total Time _____

Max VO$_2$ _____METS _____ Type of Test _____

Recommendation for exercise. MODERATE is defined as standing, walking, bending, reaching and light exercise 3 days a week. Please *check* one:

__There is no contraindication to participation in a MODERATE exercise program.
__Because of the above analysis, participation in a MODERATE exercise program may be advisable, but further examination or consultation is necessary, namely: STRESS TEST, EKG, OTHER _____
__Because of the above analysis, my patient may participate only under direct supervision of a physician. (CARDIAC REHABILITATION PROGRAM)
__Because of the above analysis, participation in a MODERATE exercise program is inadvisable.

C. SUMMARY IMPRESSION OF PHYSICIAN

    1. Comments on any history of orthopedic and neuromuscular disorders that may affect participation in an exercise program—especially those checked.

_____

    2. Message for the Exercise Program Director: _____

_____

Physician: _____ Signature: _____
             (Please type/print)
Address: _____ Phone:_( ) _____

PART III — PATIENT'S RELEASE AND CONSENT

__RELEASE: I hereby release the above information to the Exercise Director.
__CONSENT: I agree to see my private physician for medical care and agree to have an evaluation by him/her once a year if necessary.

SIGNED: _____ Date: _____

9   Guidelines for Exercise Programs for Persons 60 Years and Older

It is generally accepted that exercise is beneficial to the health and well-being of the older individual. However, the type of exercise, the frequency of the exercise, the duration of the exercise and the intensity of the exercise is critical to the benefit that can be obtained. On one hand, the exercise may be so limited that it will not illicit the response that will benefit the individual. On the other hand, the exercise may be so intensive or otherwise inappropriate that it may prove harmful to the individual. It must be understood that these guidelines simply provide guidance to those who administer or develop exercise programs for older adults. Each situation has its won uniqueness which also must be taken into consideration.

General Guidelines

1. The exercise programs should be tailored to the individual's functional capacity and should be preceded by the following:

    a. Evaluation of medical history and present status.

    b. An evaluation of functional capacity as related to physical capabilities.

2. The evaluation should include measures similar to those included in the exercise program.

3. The results of the evaluation should be used to develop an exercise prescription that includes the type, frequency, duration and intensity of the exercise.

4. The exercise leader should understand the visible signs of exhaustion and always be in a position to observe these signs.

5. The number of individuals in a given exercise group should not be larger than that which will allow constant personal contact with the instructor.

6. The instructor should be capable of handling emergency care procedures and have an emergency plan that includes response services within a reasonable period of time.

7.   The instructor should insure that clothing worn is appropriate to maintain proper body temperature and insure that water is replaced according to the amount of water lost through exercise.

8.   The exercise program should have a set of written objectives that relate to the exercise prescription and the desired outcomes for the group involved.

9.   The facilities used should be free of obstacles and have a non-slippery floor surface that does not predispose participants to lower body injury. (i.e. shin splints, etc.)

10.   The exercise program should have an education component for participants that includes the following:

    a.   The proper execution of the exercises and the possible physiological and psychological effects of these exercises.

    b.   The contraindications of the exercises prescribed.

    c.   The effects of the environment, the interaction of drugs, and the effect of nutrition on the participant's response to exercise.

    d.   The importance of and the acceptable procedures that can be used to self-monitor the effects of exercise on the participant.

11.   The person developing and/or conducting the program should understand the physiological, kinesiological, and psychological implications of exercise for the older adult.

12.   If sophisticated equipment is used in the conduct of the program, instructions for the proper use of that equipment should be given to each participant and posted for continued reference as the equipment is being used.

Guidelines for Low Intensity Exercise

This section relates to exercise that is consistent with activities of daily living for the group involved and for individuals that are apparently healthy. These individuals are not being treated regularly by a physician.

1.   Consent of the medical doctor is recommended, but not required.

2.   The program should include a wide range of activities which include aerobic, flexibility/mobility, resistance and fine motor components.

3.   Care should be taken to maintain the stability of the individuals involved to avoid loss of balance or equilibrium.

42

4. The intensity of the program should be monitored and related to the functional capacity of the participant.

Guidelines for Higher Intensity Exercise

This section relates to exercise beyond the limits of daily living for the group involved or those being treated by a physician.

1. Consent of medical doctor is required with approval related to the prescription for exercise to be used.
2. The intensity of the exercise should be monitored on a regular basis. Heart rate and/or perceived exertion are suggested as measures and should be related to the functional capacity of the participant. Accepted target heart rate tables or formulas should be used to determine intensity levels.
3. The program should include a warm up and a cool down in addition to the regular workout.
4. The program should start well below functional capacity and demonstrate reasonable progression of intensity over time.
5. The instructor should have a written list of symptoms of exhaustion and/or overexertion that are readily available and understood.

10 Suggested Resources

1.   Adrian, M.J. (1981). Flexibility In The Aging Adult. In E.L. Smith and R.C. Serfass (Eds.). *Exercise and Aging: The Scientific Basis.* Hillside, NJ: Enslow Publishers. 45-47.

2.   American College of Sports Medicine. (1991). *Guidelines for exercise testing and prescription* (4th ed.). Philadelphia: Lea & Febiger.

3.   Bazzano, C., Cunningham, L., Cama, G., & Falconio, T. (1995). Physiology of the 1-Mile Walk Test in Older Adults. *Journal of Aging and Physical Activity,* 3:4, 373-382.

4.   Besdine, R.W., Wakefield, K.M., & Williams, T.F. (1988). Assessing function in the elderly. *Patient Care,* 22, 69-79.

5.   Bookwalter, K.W. (1950). Grip Strength Norms For Males. *Research Quarterly* 21. 249-273.

6.   Cole, J.J., & Abbs, J.H. (1986). Coordination of three-joint digit movements for rapid finger-thumb grasp. *Journal of Neurophysiology,* 55, 1407-1423.

7.   Deniston, O.L., & Jette, A. (1980). A functional status assessment instrument: Validation in an elderly population. *Health Services Research,* 15, 21-34.

8.   Elam, J.T., Graney, M.J., Beaver, T., Derwi, D.E., Applegate, W.B. & Miller, S.T. (1991). Comparison of subjective ratings of function with observed functional ability of frail older persons. *American Journal of Public Health,* 81, 1127-1130.

9.   Evans, B., Hopkins, D., & Toney, T. (1996). Metabolic Response to the Half- Mile AAHPERD Functional Fitness Walk Test in Older Adults. *Journal of Aging and Physical Activity,* 4:1, 80-89.

10.   Gerety, M.B., Mulrow, M.R. Huzuda, H., Lichtenstein, J.M., O'Neil, M., Gorton, A., & Bohannon, R. (1993). Development and validation of a physical performance instrument for the functionally impaired elderly: The physical Disability Index (PDI). *Journal of Gerontology: Medical Sciences,* 48, M33-M38.

11.   Gromak, P.A., & Waskel, S.A. (1989). Functional assessment in the elderly: A literature review. *Physical and Occupational Therapy in Geriatrics,* 7, 1-12.

12. Hodgson, J.L. & Buskirk, E.R. (1977). Physical Fitness And Age, With Emphasis On Cardiovascular Function In The Elderly. *Journal of American Geriatric Society* 25, 385-392.

13. Leaf, D., & MacRae, H. (1995). Validity of Two Indirect Measures of Energy Expenditure During Walking in the Elderly. *Journal of Aging and Physical Activity.* 3:1, 97-106.

14. Lemsky, C., Miller, C.J., Nevitt, M., & Winograd, C. (1991). Reliability and validity of a physical performance and mobility examination for hospitalized elderly. *Society of Gerontology (Abstracts)*, 31, 221.

15. Londeree, B.R. & Moeschberger, M.L. (1982). Effect Of Age And Other Factors On Maximal Heart Rate. *Research Quarterly For Exercise and Sports,* 53, 297-304.

16. Osness, W.H. (1987). Assessment of physical function among older adults. In D. Leslie (Ed.), *Mature Stuff.* Reston, VA: American Association for Health, Physical Education, Recreation and Dance.

17. Osness, W.H. (1989). Assessment Of Physical Function Among OlderAdults. *Mature Stuff,* AAHPERD Publications, 93-115.

18. Osness, W.H. (March, 1989). AAHPERD Fitness Task Force: History And Philosophy. JOPERD, 64-65.

19. Reuben, D.B., & Siu, A.L. (1990). An objective measure of Physical function of elderly outpatients: The physical performance test. *Journal of the American Geriatrics Society,* 38, 1105-1112.

20. Shanlis, D., Golding, L., & Tandy, R. (1994). Reliability of the AAHPERD Functional Fitness Assessment Across Multiple Practice Sessions in Older Men and Women. *Journal of Aging and Physical Activity,* 2:3, 237-279.

21. Shiffman, L.M. (1992). Effects of aging on adult hand function. *American Journal of Occupational Therapy,* 46, 785-792.

22. Tinetti, M.E. (1986), Performance-oriented assessment of mobility problems in elderly patients. *Journal of the American Geriatrics Society ,* 34, 119-126.

23. Warren, B., Dotson, R., Nieman, D., & Butterworth, D. (1993) Validation of a 1-Mile Walk Test in Elderly Women, *Journal of Aging and Physical Activity,* 1:1, 13-21.

24. Williams, J.H., Drinka, T.J.K., Greenberg, J.R., Farrell-Holtan, J., Euhardy, R., & Schram, M. (1991). Development and testing of the Assessment of Living Skills and Resources (ALSAR) in elderly community-dwelling veterans. *The Gerontologist,* 31, 84-91.

NEW! COMPANION TO THE TEST MANUAL

New this year is a video tape to help you learn the protocol for administering the *Functional Fitness Assessment for Adults Over 60 Years*. Dr. Osness takes you step by step through each test item with demonstration of how each item is performed and tips on what to look for with various conditions. Using this video will help you quickly learn the administration procedures and unlike a workshop, can be re-played again and again. Stock # 302-10035. To order *Administering the Functional Fitness Assessment*, call: AAHPERD Publications (800) 321-0789 or FAX your order to: (301) 567-9553. A purchase order may be mailed to: AAHPERD Publications, P.O. Box 385, Oxon Hill, MD 20750-0385.

OTHER BOOKS BY CAAD

Elder Fit: A Health and Fitness Guide for Older Adults

A comprehensive exercise and fitness program for frail elderly with eight pre-planned exercise sessions. Stock #A475-1

Exercise and the Older Adult

This is the prime textbook in the field including biomechanics, exercise physiology and motor learning of aging. Activity planning includes sitting as well as aquatic exercise and dance. Stock # 302-10037

Research Sourcebook and Bibliography in Aging and Health, Exercise, Recreation and Dance

A ready-made bibliography of current publications in exercise and aging. It also includes listings of private foundations and other funding sources. Stock # 302-10003

Maximizing Options for a Quality Life

This informative pamphlet represents CAAD's position on the professional standards that should be met by facilities offering programs for seniors. Stock # 302-10034

Guidelines for Exercise Programs for Persons 60 Years and Older

The same guidelines contained in this manual can be purchased for distribution in quantity. Stock # 302-10036

Fitness Programs for Older Adults: A Leadership Training Workshop

Watch for this two-day workshop offered at various sites around the country. Training for practitioners includes chronic conditions and contraindications for exercise, frail elderly assessment and exercise, aquatic exercise, well elderly and exercise, functional fitness assessment, Tai Chi and more. For more information on the workshop next scheduled workshop call: (800) 213-7193 x430.

COUNCIL ON AGING AND ADULT
DEVELOPMENT PURPOSE

The Council on Aging and Adult Development (CAAD) is one of the most active Councils in our nation promoting quality life experiences for older adults through physical activity. As one of the Councils of the American Association for Active Lifestyles and Fitness (AAALF), CAAD works to encourage professional services to the elderly by way of leadership, research and programs in the fields of health, physical education, recreation and dance.

CAAD members have been instrumental in developing guidelines for programs designed to meet the needs of older adults. Some older adults who have been active all their lives remain so well into their senior years. Others, because of lifestyle changes or medical conditions are unable to continue to pursue their activity interests or wish to pursue new ones. All too frequently, medical conditions demand that physical activity become a part of a person's lifestyle and professional guidance and sometimes monitoring is necessary for safe and successful participation. CAAD is comprised of professionals who practice, teach and/or have devised the standard of professional practice for the older adult in the physical activity arena.

Research forms the foundation for program content and CAAD has provided leadership in this area as well. Until 1990 when the first edition of this manual was published, no guideline for assessment of the older adult in the area of motor performance existed. Only medical evaluation was available to determine if individuals were "fit" to begin an exercise program. After five long years of dedicated service, CAAD members, lead by Dr. Wayne Osness of the University of Kansas, trained individuals to administer this test and gather data to use in developing the norms contained in this edition. This test measures the performances needed to meet the practical demands of daily living and should form the basis for at least part of an exercise program for this population.

A variety of programs fill CAAD's agenda including publications containing activity ideas and foundation materials for people preparing to work with the older population. CAAD's leadership training workshop is becoming well-known as the best two day training for the practitioner already in the field. Advocacy is another program continually at the forefront of CAAD's activities including participation in the White House Conference on Aging in 1995 with notable impact on resolutions related to health care and quality of life issues.

For more information on CAAD and its activities call the AAALF headquarters at: (800) 213-7193.